Blood Type O Diet and Meal Plan

Delicious and Easy Recipes to Optimal Health, Energy, and Weight Loss for Blood Type O Positive and O Negative

Rosalee Casper

Table of Contents

Introduction

Understanding Blood Type O

Blood type is determined by the presence or absence of specific antigens on the surface of red blood cells. The ABO blood group system categorizes individuals into four main types: A, B, AB, and O. Blood Type O is characterized by the absence of A and B antigens, making it the universal blood donor type. Genetic inheritance plays a crucial role in determining an individual's blood type, with each parent contributing one allele to their offspring.

Individuals with Blood Type O possess distinct physiological characteristics that set them apart from other blood types. They are often described as having a robust immune system and a strong, resilient digestive system. Blood Type O individuals tend to thrive on high-protein diets and vigorous physical activity. Moreover, they exhibit traits such as being goal-oriented, practical, and adaptable, which influence their lifestyle preferences and dietary needs.

Research suggests that blood type may influence susceptibility to certain health conditions and diseases. Blood Type O individuals may have a lower risk of developing heart disease and certain types of cancer compared to individuals with other blood types. However, they may be more prone to certain digestive issues, such as ulcers and stomach sensitivities. Understanding these health implications is essential for tailoring a diet and lifestyle that promotes optimal health and well-being for Blood Type O individuals.

Importance of Following a Blood Type O Meal Plan

Optimizing Nutrient Intake

Following a Blood Type O meal plan ensures that individuals with Blood Type O receive optimal nutrient intake tailored to their specific genetic makeup and physiological characteristics. By focusing on foods that are compatible with the Blood Type O profile, such as lean proteins, vegetables, and fruits, while limiting or avoiding foods that may be less beneficial, individuals can maximize nutrient absorption and support overall health and well-being.

Enhancing Digestive Function

The Blood Type O meal plan emphasizes foods that are easily digestible and less likely to cause digestive discomfort or inflammation for individuals with Blood Type O. By minimizing the consumption of grains, dairy, and legumes, which may be less compatible with the digestive enzymes of Blood Type O individuals, the meal plan promotes better digestive function and reduces the risk of gastrointestinal issues such as bloating, gas, and indigestion.

Supporting Weight Management Goals

For individuals with Blood Type O who are looking to manage their weight effectively, following a structured meal plan can be instrumental in achieving their goals. The Blood Type O meal plan emphasizes nutrient-dense foods that provide sustained energy and promote satiety, helping individuals feel satisfied and reducing the likelihood of overeating or reaching for unhealthy snacks. Additionally, the emphasis on lean proteins and vegetables can support muscle maintenance and metabolism, contributing to a healthy body composition.

Promoting Overall Health and Well-being

Beyond weight management, following a Blood Type O meal plan is essential for promoting overall health and well-being. By aligning dietary choices with the genetic predispositions and physiological characteristics of Blood Type O individuals, the meal plan can help optimize immune function, enhance energy levels, and reduce the risk of chronic diseases such as heart disease and certain types of cancer. Moreover, by fostering a balanced and sustainable approach to nutrition, the meal plan supports long-term health outcomes and improves quality of life for individuals with Blood Type O.

Chapter 1: The Science behind Blood Type O

Genetics and Blood Type

The ABO blood group system is one of the most well-known classification systems for human blood types. It categorizes individuals into four main blood types: A, B, AB, and O. These blood types are determined by the presence or absence of specific antigens on the surface of red blood cells. For example, individuals with Blood Type A have A antigens, those with Blood Type B have B antigens, those with Blood Type AB have both A and B antigens, and those with Blood Type O lack A and B antigens.

The inheritance of blood type follows Mendelian principles, with each individual inheriting one allele from each parent. The ABO gene, located on chromosome 9, encodes the enzymes responsible for the production of A and B antigens. The presence or absence of these antigens is determined by variations in the ABO gene alleles. For example, individuals with two A alleles (AA genotype) will have Blood Type A, while those with two B alleles (BB genotype) will have Blood Type B. Individuals with one A allele and one B allele (AB genotype) will have Blood Type

AB, and those with two O alleles (OO genotype) will have Blood Type O.

Characteristics of Blood Type O Individuals

Physiological Traits

Blood Type O individuals possess several physiological traits that set them apart from individuals with other blood types. They often have a robust immune system, characterized by a strong response to infections and a lower susceptibility to certain diseases. Additionally, Blood Type O individuals tend to have a more efficient metabolism, which may contribute to their ability to process and metabolize food more effectively.

Personality Tendencies

Research suggests that blood type may be linked to certain personality traits and tendencies. Blood Type O individuals are often described as being practical, goal-oriented, and assertive. They tend to be natural leaders, with a strong sense of responsibility and a desire for success. Moreover, Blood Type O individuals are known for their adaptability and resilience, allowing them to navigate challenging situations with ease.

Dietary Considerations

The characteristics of Blood Type O individuals also influence their dietary needs and preferences. Due to their efficient metabolism and active lifestyle, Blood Type O individuals typically thrive on a diet rich in lean proteins, fruits, and vegetables. They may benefit from higher protein intake to support muscle growth and energy levels, as well as an emphasis on whole, nutrient-dense foods to support overall health and well-being.

Exercise Recommendations

Blood Type O individuals are often drawn to vigorous physical activity and may excel in sports and fitness pursuits. Their natural athleticism and endurance make them well-suited for activities such as running, weightlifting, and martial arts. Incorporating regular exercise into their routine can help Blood Type O individuals maintain optimal health, manage stress, and enhance overall fitness levels.

Lower Risk of Heart Disease

Research suggests that individuals with Blood Type O may have a lower risk of developing heart disease compared to individuals with other blood types. This protective effect is thought to be related to certain physiological characteristics associated with Blood Type O, such as lower levels of blood clotting factors and reduced risk of thrombosis. Additionally, the Blood Type O diet, which emphasizes lean proteins and avoids certain foods that may contribute to heart disease risk, may further reduce the risk of cardiovascular issues for Blood Type O individuals.

Reduced Risk of Certain Cancers

In addition to heart disease, Blood Type O individuals may also have a lower risk of developing certain types of cancer, including pancreatic cancer and stomach cancer. Research has suggested that individuals with Blood Type O may have a reduced susceptibility to certain carcinogens and toxins, as well as a more robust immune response to cancer cells. However, further studies are needed to fully understand the mechanisms underlying this association.

Higher Susceptibility to Stomach Sensitivities

Despite the potential health advantages associated with Blood Type O, individuals with this blood type may be more susceptible to certain digestive issues, such as stomach sensitivities and ulcers. Research has indicated that individuals with Blood Type O may produce higher levels of stomach acid, which can increase the risk of gastrointestinal issues such as acid reflux and gastritis. It's important for Blood Type O individuals to be mindful of their digestive health and to adopt dietary and lifestyle habits that support optimal gastrointestinal function.

Potential Impact on Fertility and Reproductive Health

Some research suggests that blood type may influence fertility and reproductive health outcomes. While the evidence is still emerging, there is some evidence to suggest that individuals with Blood Type O may have a higher risk of certain reproductive disorders, such as ovarian dysfunction and endometriosis. However, more research is needed to fully understand the relationship between blood type and reproductive health.

Chapter 2: Foundations of the Blood Type O Diet

Principles of the Blood Type O Diet

Emphasis on Protein-Rich Foods

One of the central principles of the Blood Type O diet is the emphasis on consuming protein-rich foods, particularly lean sources of animal protein. This includes poultry, fish, and red meat, which provide essential nutrients such as iron, zinc, and B vitamins. Protein is essential for muscle growth and repair, energy production, and overall metabolic function, making it a cornerstone of the Blood Type O diet.

Limitation of Grains, Dairy, and Legumes

In contrast to other blood types, individuals with Blood Type O are advised to limit or avoid certain foods that may be less compatible with their genetic makeup and digestive enzymes. This includes grains, dairy products, and legumes, which are believed to be less beneficial for Blood Type O individuals. These foods may contribute to digestive issues, inflammation, and other health concerns, making it important to minimize their consumption in the Blood Type O diet.

Focus on Whole, Nutrient-Dense Foods

Another key principle of the Blood Type O diet is the focus on whole, nutrient-dense foods that provide essential vitamins, minerals, and antioxidants. This includes a variety of fruits and vegetables, which are rich in fiber, vitamins, and phytonutrients that support overall health and well-being. By prioritizing these foods, individuals with Blood Type O can ensure they are meeting their nutritional needs while supporting optimal digestion and metabolic function.

Foods to Embrace and Avoid

Embrace: Lean Proteins

One of the key food groups that individuals with Blood Type O are encouraged to embrace is lean proteins. This includes poultry such as chicken and turkey, fish such as salmon and cod, and red meat such as beef and lamb. These protein-rich foods provide essential nutrients such as iron, zinc, and B vitamins, which are important for muscle growth, energy production, and overall metabolic function.

Embrace: Fruits and Vegetables

Another important component of the Blood Type O diet is fruits and vegetables. These nutrient-dense foods are rich in vitamins, minerals, and antioxidants that support overall health and well-being. Blood Type O individuals are encouraged to consume a variety of fruits and vegetables, including leafy greens, berries, citrus fruits, and cruciferous vegetables such as broccoli and Brussels sprouts.

Embrace: Healthy Fats

While individuals with Blood Type O are encouraged to limit their intake of certain fats, such as saturated fats found in red meat and dairy products, they can still include healthy fats in their diet. This includes sources such as olive oil, avocados, nuts, and seeds, which provide essential fatty acids that support heart health, brain function, and overall well-being.

Avoid: Grains

One category of foods that individuals with Blood Type O are advised to avoid or limit is grains. This includes wheat, barley, rye, and products made from these grains, such as bread, pasta, and cereal. Grains are believed to be less compatible with the digestive enzymes of Blood Type O individuals and may contribute to digestive issues and inflammation.

Avoid: Dairy Products

Similarly, dairy products are generally not recommended for individuals with Blood Type O. This includes milk, cheese, yogurt, and other dairy-based products. Dairy products may be more difficult for Blood Type O individuals to digest and may contribute to digestive discomfort and other health issues.

Avoid: Legumes

Legumes such as beans, lentils, and soy products are also advised to be limited or avoided in the Blood Type O diet. While legumes are a good source of plant-based protein and fiber, they may be less compatible with the digestive enzymes of Blood Type O individuals and may contribute to digestive issues such as gas and bloating.

Chapter 3: Planning Your Blood Type O Meals

Meal Planning Basics

Understanding Your Dietary Requirements

The first step in meal planning for Blood Type O individuals is to understand their specific dietary requirements and preferences. This includes considering their protein needs, carbohydrate tolerance, and preferences for certain foods and flavors. By taking stock of their nutritional needs and personal preferences, individuals can tailor their meal plans to align with their goals and lifestyle.

Creating Balanced Meals

A balanced meal for Blood Type O individuals typically includes a lean source of protein, plenty of fruits and vegetables, and a moderate amount of healthy fats. When planning meals, aim to include a variety of colors, textures, and flavors to ensure a well-rounded and satisfying dining experience. Additionally, consider incorporating a mix of macronutrients, including protein, carbohydrates, and fats, to support optimal energy levels and metabolic function.

Meal Prepping for Success

Meal prepping is a valuable tool for Blood Type O individuals looking to streamline their meal planning process and simplify their daily routine. Set aside time each week to plan and prepare meals in advance, taking into account your schedule, dietary preferences, and nutritional needs. Batch cooking staple ingredients such as proteins, grains, and vegetables can save time and effort during busy weekdays, making it easier to stick to your dietary goals.

Incorporating Variety and Flexibility

While meal planning provides structure and guidance, it's important to maintain flexibility and incorporate variety into your diet. Experiment with different recipes, ingredients, and cuisines to keep meals interesting and enjoyable. Additionally, listen to your body's cues and adjust your meal plan as needed based on changes in appetite, energy levels, and preferences.

Mindful Eating Practices

In addition to planning and preparing meals, practicing mindful eating can enhance your overall dining experience and promote a greater connection with your food. Take time to savor each bite, chew slowly, and pay attention to hunger and fullness cues. Mindful eating can help prevent overeating, improve digestion, and foster a deeper appreciation for the nourishing properties of food.

Sample Meal Plans for Different Lifestyles

Meal Plan for Busy Professionals

Breakfast

- Greek yogurt with mixed berries and almonds
- Green tea

Lunch

- Grilled chicken salad with mixed greens, cherry tomatoes, cucumbers, and avocado
- Olive oil and lemon dressing

Snack

- Sliced apple with almond butter

Dinner

- Baked salmon with roasted asparagus and quinoa
- Herbal tea

Meal Plan for Busy Families

Breakfast

- Omelette with spinach, tomatoes, and feta cheese
- Whole grain toast with avocado

Lunch

- Turkey and cheese whole grain wraps with mixed greens and bell peppers
- Carrot sticks with hummus

Snack

- Greek yogurt with honey and granola

Dinner

- Beef stir-fry with broccoli, bell peppers, and brown rice
- Fruit salad with berries and melon

Meal Plan for Athletes

Breakfast

- Protein smoothie with banana, spinach, almond milk, and protein powder
- Whole grain toast with peanut butter

Lunch

- Grilled chicken breast with sweet potato and steamed broccoli
- Mixed green salad with balsamic vinaigrette

Snack

- Cottage cheese with pineapple chunks

Dinner

- Lean beef steak with quinoa and roasted vegetables
- Greek salad with feta cheese, olives, and tomatoes

Chapter 4: Breakfast Recipes

Protein-Packed Parfait

Preparation Time:	10 minutes

Ingredients

- 1 cup Greek yogurt (preferably full-fat)
- 1/4 cup mixed nuts (such as almonds, walnuts, and pecans), chopped
- 2 tablespoons seeds (such as chia seeds, hemp seeds, or flaxseeds)
- 1/2 cup mixed berries (such as strawberries, blueberries, and raspberries), fresh or frozen
- 1/4 cup granola (choose a Blood Type O-friendly option or make your own)
- Honey or maple syrup (optional, for sweetness)

Instructions

1.
   - If using frozen berries, place them in a small saucepan over medium heat. If using fresh berries, you can skip this step.
   - Cook the berries, stirring occasionally, until they release their juices and start to break down, about 5-7 minutes.

	• Remove from heat and let cool slightly. You can sweeten the compote with a drizzle of honey or maple syrup if desired. Allow to cool completely.
2	• In serving glasses or jars, start by adding a layer of Greek yogurt to the bottom of each. • Next, sprinkle a layer of chopped nuts over the yogurt. • Add a layer of seeds on top of the nuts. • Spoon a layer of the berry compote over the seeds. • Repeat the layers until the glasses or jars are filled, ending with a final layer of yogurt on top.
3	• Finish off each parfait by sprinkling a generous amount of granola on top of the yogurt layer. • Optionally, drizzle with a little extra honey or maple syrup for added sweetness.
4	Serve the protein-packed parfaits immediately for a delicious and energizing morning treat.

Savory Breakfast Grain Bowl

Preparation Time:	15 minutes

Ingredients

- 1 cup cooked quinoa or brown rice
- 2 large eggs
- 1 cup mixed greens (such as spinach, kale, or Swiss chard)
- 1/2 avocado, sliced
- 1 tablespoon tahini or hot sauce (optional, for drizzling)
- Salt and pepper to taste
- Olive oil for cooking

Instructions

1	If you haven't already cooked the quinoa or brown rice, prepare it according to package instructions. Once cooked, set aside.
2	<ul><li>Bring a medium pot of water to a gentle simmer over medium heat.</li><li>Crack the eggs into individual small bowls or ramekins.</li><li>Carefully slide each egg into the simmering water, one at a time.</li></ul>

	<ul><li>Cook the eggs for about 3-4 minutes, or until the whites are set but the yolks are still runny.</li><li>Use a slotted spoon to carefully remove the poached eggs from the water and set them aside.</li></ul>
3	<ul><li>In a skillet, heat a drizzle of olive oil over medium heat.</li><li>Add the mixed greens to the skillet and sauté until wilted, about 2-3 minutes.</li><li>Season the greens with salt and pepper to taste.</li></ul>
4	<ul><li>Divide the cooked quinoa or brown rice between two bowls.</li><li>Top each bowl with the sautéed greens, sliced avocado, and a poached egg.</li><li>Drizzle with tahini or hot sauce, if using, for added flavor and protein.</li></ul>
5	<ul><li>Serve the savory breakfast grain bowls immediately while still warm.</li><li>Season with additional salt and pepper if desired.</li></ul>

Nourishing Smoothie Bowl

Preparation Time:	10 minutes

Ingredients

For the Smoothie Base:

- 1 frozen banana, sliced
- 1/2 cup frozen berries (such as strawberries, blueberries, or raspberries)
- 1 cup fresh spinach or kale leaves
- 1/2 cup unsweetened almond milk or coconut water
- 1 tablespoon chia seeds or flaxseeds
- 1 tablespoon almond butter or peanut butter (optional, for added creaminess)
- 1 teaspoon honey or maple syrup (optional, for sweetness)
- 1/2 teaspoon matcha powder or acai powder (optional, for additional nutrients and flavor)

For Toppings:

- Chia seeds
- Hemp hearts
- Sliced almonds
- Fresh berries (such as strawberries, blueberries, or raspberries)

- Shredded coconut
- Granola or muesli

Instructions

1	- In a blender, combine the frozen banana, frozen berries, fresh spinach or kale leaves, almond milk or coconut water, chia seeds or flaxseeds, almond butter or peanut butter (if using), honey or maple syrup (if using), and matcha powder or acai powder (if using). - Blend until smooth and creamy, adding more liquid if needed to reach your desired consistency.
2	- Pour the smoothie into a bowl. - Top with a variety of superfood toppings such as chia seeds, hemp hearts, sliced almonds, fresh berries, shredded coconut, and granola or muesli.
3	Get creative with your smoothie bowl by experimenting with unexpected flavor combinations. Try mixing acai powder with kale for a vibrant green bowl, or blend matcha powder with pineapple for a refreshing twist.
4	Serve the nourishing smoothie bowl immediately.

Seaweed Breakfast Wrap

Preparation Time:	15 minutes

Ingredients

- 4 sheets of nori seaweed
- 4 large eggs
- 4 ounces smoked salmon
- 1 ripe avocado, sliced
- 1 small cucumber, julienned
- Soy sauce or tamari (optional, for serving)
- Sesame seeds (optional, for garnish)
- Olive oil or cooking spray

Instructions

1.
   - In a bowl, whisk together the eggs until well beaten.
   - Heat a skillet over medium heat and lightly coat with olive oil or cooking spray.
   - Pour the beaten eggs into the skillet and cook, stirring occasionally, until scrambled and cooked through. Remove from heat and set aside.

2.
   - Lay a sheet of nori seaweed on a clean, dry surface.

- Place a portion of scrambled eggs in the center of the seaweed sheet, leaving some space around the edges.

- Arrange slices of smoked salmon, avocado, and julienned cucumber on top of the scrambled eggs.

3
- Starting from one edge, carefully roll the seaweed sheet around the filling ingredients, using your fingers to tuck in the sides as you roll.

- Continue rolling until the seaweed forms a tight wrap around the filling.

- Repeat with the remaining seaweed sheets and filling ingredients.

4
- Use a sharp knife to slice each seaweed wrap in half or into smaller pieces, if desired.

- Serve the seaweed breakfast wraps immediately, with soy sauce or tamari on the side for dipping, if desired.

- Garnish with sesame seeds for added flavor and texture, if desired.

Quick Breakfast Quesadillas

Preparation Time:	15 minutes

Ingredients

- 4 whole grain tortillas
- 4 large eggs
- 1/2 cup black beans, drained and rinsed
- 1/2 cup diced bell peppers (any color)
- 1/2 cup shredded cheese (such as cheddar, Monterey Jack, or Mexican blend)
- Salt and pepper to taste
- Cooking spray or olive oil
- Salsa or Greek yogurt for serving (optional)

Instructions

1	• In a bowl, whisk together the eggs until well beaten. Season with salt and pepper to taste. • Heat a skillet over medium heat and lightly coat with cooking spray or olive oil. • Pour the beaten eggs into the skillet and cook, stirring occasionally, until scrambled and cooked through. Remove from heat and set aside.
2	• Lay out the whole grain tortillas on a clean, dry surface.

	• Divide the scrambled eggs, black beans, diced bell peppers, and shredded cheese evenly among the tortillas, placing the fillings on one half of each tortilla.
3	• Fold the empty half of each tortilla over the filling to create a half-moon shape. • Heat a large skillet or griddle over medium heat. Lightly coat with cooking spray or olive oil. • Place the assembled quesadillas in the skillet and cook for 2-3 minutes on each side, or until golden brown and crispy, and the cheese is melted.
4	• Remove the cooked quesadillas from the skillet and transfer to a cutting board. • Use a sharp knife to cut each quesadilla into wedges. • Serve the breakfast quesadillas immediately, with salsa or Greek yogurt for dipping if desired.

DIY Breakfast Sushi Rolls

Preparation Time:	15 minutes

Ingredients

- 2 nori seaweed sheets
- 4 large eggs
- 1 avocado, sliced
- 4 ounces smoked salmon or cooked shrimp
- Cooked sushi rice or regular rice (optional)
- Soy sauce or tamari, for dipping (optional)
- Pickled ginger and wasabi, for serving (optional)

Instructions

1.
   - Cook the eggs: In a bowl, whisk together the eggs until well beaten. Heat a skillet over medium heat and lightly coat with cooking spray or olive oil. Pour the beaten eggs into the skillet and cook, stirring occasionally, until scrambled and cooked through. Remove from heat and set aside.
   - Slice the avocado: Cut the avocado in half, remove the pit, and slice the avocado into thin strips. Set aside.
   - Prepare the smoked salmon or cooked shrimp: If using smoked salmon, slice it into thin strips.

		If using cooked shrimp, ensure they are peeled, deveined, and sliced in half lengthwise. Set aside.
2	•	Place a nori seaweed sheet on a clean, dry surface, with the shiny side facing down.
	•	If using sushi rice or regular rice, spread a thin layer of rice evenly over the nori sheet, leaving about 1 inch of space at the top edge.
	•	Arrange the scrambled eggs, sliced avocado, and smoked salmon or cooked shrimp in a line across the bottom edge of the nori sheet.
3	•	Starting from the bottom edge, tightly roll up the nori sheet, using your fingers to press down gently to seal the edge.
	•	Continue rolling until you reach the top edge of the nori sheet.
	•	Use a sharp knife to slice the sushi roll into bite-sized pieces, about 1 inch wide.
4	•	Arrange the DIY breakfast sushi rolls on a plate and serve immediately.
	•	If desired, serve with soy sauce or tamari for dipping, and offer pickled ginger and wasabi on the side for added flavor.

DIY Breakfast Bento Boxes

Preparation Time:	15 minutes

Ingredients

- Hard-boiled eggs
- Mixed nuts (such as almonds, walnuts, and cashews)
- Sliced fruit (such as apples, bananas, and berries)
- Whole grain crackers or rice cakes
- Other optional additions: sliced vegetables (such as carrots, cucumber, and bell peppers), hummus, Greek yogurt, cheese slices, turkey or chicken slices, nut butter packets, granola or muesli, dried fruit (such as apricots or raisins)

Instructions

1.
   - Place the desired number of eggs in a pot and cover them with cold water.
   - Bring the water to a boil over medium-high heat, then reduce the heat to low and simmer for 10-12 minutes.
   - Remove the eggs from the pot and transfer them to a bowl of ice water to cool. Once cooled, peel the eggs and set them aside.

2	• Divide the hard-boiled eggs, mixed nuts, sliced fruit, and whole grain crackers or rice cakes among the compartments of your bento boxes. • Arrange the items in each compartment in a visually appealing manner, ensuring there is a balance of protein, healthy fats, carbohydrates, and fiber.
3	• Get creative and customize your bento boxes with additional ingredients according to your preferences and dietary needs. • Add sliced vegetables and hummus for extra fiber and nutrients. • Include Greek yogurt topped with granola or muesli for a creamy and crunchy addition. • Add cheese slices and turkey or chicken slices for additional protein. • Include nut butter packets for spreading on whole grain crackers or rice cakes. • Add dried fruit for a sweet and chewy snack option.
4	Once assembled, securely close the lids of your bento boxes and store them in the refrigerator until ready to eat.

Microwave Mug Oatmeal

Preparation Time:	2 minutes

Ingredients

- 1/3 cup rolled oats
- 2/3 cup water or milk of choice
- Pinch of salt
- Optional add-ins: sliced banana, berries, nuts, seeds, honey, maple syrup, cinnamon

Instructions

1	In a microwave-safe mug, combine the rolled oats, water or milk, and a pinch of salt.
2	Microwave on high for 1 minute.
3	Stir the oatmeal, then microwave for an additional 1-2 minutes, stirring every 30 seconds, until the oatmeal is cooked to your desired consistency.
4	Add any desired toppings such as sliced banana, berries, nuts, seeds, honey, maple syrup, or cinnamon.
5	Stir to combine and enjoy your warm and comforting microwave mug oatmeal.

Chapter 5: Lunch Recipes

Mediterranean Quinoa Salad

Preparation Time:	20 minutes

Ingredients

- 1 cup quinoa, rinsed and cooked
- 1 cucumber, diced
- 1 pint cherry tomatoes, halved
- 1/2 red onion, thinly sliced
- 1/2 cup Kalamata olives, pitted and halved
- 1/4 cup crumbled feta cheese
- 1/4 cup chopped fresh parsley
- Juice of 1 lemon
- 2 tablespoons extra virgin olive oil
- Salt and pepper to taste

Instructions

1. In a large bowl, combine the cooked quinoa, diced cucumber, halved cherry tomatoes, sliced red onion, halved Kalamata olives, crumbled feta cheese, and chopped parsley.

2. In a small bowl, whisk together the lemon juice, extra virgin olive oil, salt, and pepper.

| 3 | Pour the dressing over the quinoa salad and toss to combine. |
| 4 | Serve immediately or refrigerate until ready to serve. |

Deconstructed Sushi Bowl

| Preparation Time: | 20 minutes (not including rice cooking time) |

Ingredients

- 1 cup sushi rice or cauliflower rice
- 4 ounces raw or marinated fish (such as sushi-grade tuna or salmon)
- 1/2 cup seaweed salad
- 1/4 cup pickled vegetables (such as cucumber, carrot, or radish)
- 1 ripe avocado, sliced
- 2 tablespoons sesame seeds
- Soy sauce or tamari, for drizzling (optional)
- Sriracha or spicy mayo, for drizzling (optional)
- Nori strips, for garnish (optional)

Instructions

| 1 | If using sushi rice, cook according to package instructions and let it cool slightly. If using cauliflower rice, steam or sauté until tender. |

2	• Divide the cooked sushi rice or cauliflower rice among serving bowls.
	• Arrange slices of raw or marinated fish on top of the rice.
	• Add a scoop of seaweed salad to each bowl.
	• Scatter pickled vegetables and sliced avocado over the bowls.
	• Sprinkle sesame seeds over the bowls for added flavor and crunch.
3	• Drizzle soy sauce or tamari over the bowls for a traditional sushi flavor.
	• Add a drizzle of sriracha or spicy mayo for a kick of heat and creaminess.
4	• Garnish the bowls with nori strips for an extra touch of authenticity.
	• Serve the deconstructed sushi bowls immediately, allowing each person to mix the ingredients together before enjoying.

Hearty Blood Type O-Friendly Lunch Wraps

Preparation Time:	15 minutes

Ingredients

- Blood type O-friendly wraps or collard green leaves
- 8 ounces lean protein source (such as grilled chicken breast or turkey breast slices)
- 1 cup crisp vegetables (such as lettuce, shredded carrots, bell peppers, and cucumber)
- 1 ripe avocado, sliced
- Tangy sauce or spread of choice (such as hummus, tzatziki, or mustard)
- Salt and pepper to taste

Instructions

1.
   - If using collard green leaves, remove the tough stems and blanch the leaves in boiling water for 30 seconds. Pat dry with paper towels.
   - Grill or cook the lean protein source (chicken or turkey) until fully cooked. Slice into thin strips or pieces.

	• Wash and prepare crisp vegetables such as lettuce, shredded carrots, bell peppers, and cucumber.
2	• Lay a blood type O-friendly wrap or collard green leaf flat on a clean surface. • Spread a thin layer of tangy sauce or spread of choice (such as hummus, tzatziki, or mustard) over the wrap or collard green leaf. • Layer slices of grilled chicken or turkey breast on top of the sauce. • Arrange crisp vegetables and avocado slices on top of the protein layer. • Season with salt and pepper to taste.
3	• Fold in the sides of the wrap or collard green leaf, then tightly roll it up from the bottom to enclose the filling. • If using collard green leaves, tuck in the sides as you roll to keep the filling secure.
4	• Use a sharp knife to slice the wraps in half diagonally for easy serving. • Serve immediately, or wrap each half in parchment paper or foil for a convenient grab-and-go lunch option.

Crunchy Veggie Wraps

Preparation Time:	20 minutes

Ingredients

- Blood type O-friendly wraps or lettuce leaves
- Assorted julienned vegetables (such as carrots, cucumber, bell peppers, and red cabbage)
- Crispy tofu or tempeh strips
- Flavorful dipping sauce (such as peanut sauce, tahini dressing, or sweet chili sauce)
- Optional toppings: chopped fresh herbs, toasted sesame seeds, or crushed peanuts

Instructions

1.
   - Julienne the vegetables into thin strips using a sharp knife or a mandoline slicer.
   - Cut the tofu or tempeh into thin strips and pan-fry or bake until crispy.

2.
   - Lay a blood type O-friendly wrap or lettuce leaf flat on a clean work surface.
   - Arrange a handful of julienned vegetables and crispy tofu or tempeh strips in the center of the wrap or lettuce leaf.

3	<ul><li>Fold in the sides of the wrap or lettuce leaf, then tightly roll it up from the bottom to enclose the filling.</li><li>If using lettuce leaves, tuck in the sides as you roll to keep the filling secure.</li></ul>
4	<ul><li>Choose a flavorful dipping sauce such as peanut sauce, tahini dressing, or sweet chili sauce.</li><li>Serve the dipping sauce on the side in small containers for dipping.</li></ul>
5	<ul><li>Sprinkle chopped fresh herbs, toasted sesame seeds, or crushed peanuts on top of the wraps for added flavor and texture, if desired.</li><li>Serve the crunchy veggie wraps with the dipping sauce on the side for a portable and satisfying lunch option.</li></ul>

DIY Protein Box

Preparation Time:	15 minutes

Ingredients

- Hard-boiled eggs
- Cheese cubes or slices (such as cheddar, mozzarella, or Swiss)
- Mixed nuts (such as almonds, cashews, and walnuts)
- Sliced vegetables (such as carrots, cucumber, and bell peppers)
- Whole grain crackers or rice cakes
- Optional additions: hummus, Greek yogurt, fruit slices, turkey or chicken slices

Instructions

1.
   - Cook hard-boiled eggs by boiling them in water for 8-10 minutes, then cooling them in ice water before peeling.
   - Cube or slice cheese into bite-sized pieces.
   - Measure out mixed nuts or portion them into small containers.
   - Slice vegetables into sticks or rounds for easy snacking.

	• Portion whole grain crackers or rice cakes into individual servings.
2	• Use compartmentalized containers or small boxes with dividers to assemble the protein boxes. • Arrange hard-boiled eggs, cheese cubes, mixed nuts, sliced vegetables, and whole grain crackers or rice cakes in separate sections of the container. • Add optional additions such as hummus, Greek yogurt, fruit slices, or turkey or chicken slices in additional compartments if desired.
3	• Customize each protein box according to your preferences by choosing your favorite combinations of ingredients. • Pack the protein boxes in a lunch bag or cooler for a portable and customizable lunch option that's perfect for busy days.
4	Variations: • Mix and match different types of cheese, nuts, and vegetables to create a variety of flavor combinations. • Include fresh fruit slices or dried fruit for a touch of sweetness and additional nutrients.

Spiralized Veggie Salad Bowl

Preparation Time:	20 minutes

Ingredients

- Spiralized zucchini or sweet potato "noodles"
- Assorted raw or cooked vegetables (such as bell peppers, cherry tomatoes, cucumber, and avocado)
- Protein sources (such as grilled shrimp, chicken, or tofu)
- Tangy dressings (such as vinaigrette, lemon tahini dressing, or citrus avocado dressing)
- Optional toppings: chopped fresh herbs, toasted nuts or seeds, crumbled cheese or dairy-free alternative

Instructions

1.
   - Spiralize zucchini or sweet potatoes into noodles using a spiralizer or julienne peeler.
   - Wash and chop assorted raw vegetables into bite-sized pieces. If using cooked vegetables, prepare them according to your preference.
   - Cook protein sources such as shrimp, chicken, or tofu and slice them as desired.

2	<ul><li>Divide the spiralized veggie noodles among serving bowls as the base of the salad.</li><li>Arrange the assorted raw or cooked vegetables and protein sources on top of the veggie noodles.</li></ul>
3	Drizzle tangy dressings such as vinaigrette, lemon tahini dressing, or citrus avocado dressing over the salad bowls for flavor.
4	Sprinkle chopped fresh herbs, toasted nuts or seeds, or crumbled cheese or dairy-free alternative on top of the salad bowls for added texture and flavor.
5	<ul><li>Serve the spiralized veggie salad bowls immediately as a light and satisfying midday meal.</li><li>Enjoy the refreshing combination of flavors and textures in each bite, and feel free to customize the salad bowls with your favorite blood type O-friendly ingredients and dressings.</li></ul>

Vibrant Veggie Lettuce Cup

Preparation Time:	20 minutes

Ingredients

- Large lettuce leaves (such as romaine or butter lettuce)
- Seasoned ground turkey or tofu
- Shredded carrots
- Cucumber slices
- Fresh herbs (such as cilantro or mint)
- Zesty dressing or dipping sauce (such as sesame ginger dressing or sweet chili sauce)

Instructions

1
- Wash and dry the lettuce leaves, then carefully separate them and pat them dry with paper towels.
- Cook seasoned ground turkey or tofu in a skillet until browned and fully cooked.
- Shred carrots using a grater or julienne peeler.
- Slice cucumber into thin rounds.
- Wash and chop fresh herbs such as cilantro or mint.

2
- Lay the lettuce leaves flat on a clean work surface.

	• Spoon a portion of seasoned ground turkey or tofu onto each lettuce leaf.
	• Top with shredded carrots, cucumber slices, and fresh herbs.
3	• Drizzle zesty dressing or dipping sauce over the filled lettuce cups for added flavor.
	• Alternatively, serve the dressing or sauce on the side for dipping.
4	• Serve the vibrant veggie lettuce cups immediately as a colorful and crunchy lunch option.
	• Encourage diners to pick up the lettuce cups with their hands and enjoy the fresh and vibrant flavors.

Mediterranean Mezze Platter

Preparation Time:	30 minutes

Ingredients

- Hummus
- Tabbouleh
- Grilled vegetables (such as zucchini, eggplant, bell peppers, and cherry tomatoes)
- Olives (such as Kalamata or green olives)
- Feta cheese or dairy-free alternatives
- Whole grain crackers or pita bread
- Optional additions: roasted red peppers, marinated artichoke hearts, stuffed grape leaves

Instructions

1.
   - If making homemade hummus and tabbouleh, prepare them according to your favorite recipes or use store-bought versions.
   - Grill the vegetables until tender and lightly charred. Slice them into bite-sized pieces if necessary.
   - Arrange olives in a small bowl.
   - If using feta cheese, crumble it into a small bowl. If using dairy-free alternatives, prepare them according to package instructions.

2	<ul><li>Choose a large serving platter or board to arrange the mezze ingredients.</li><li>Spoon the hummus and tabbouleh into separate bowls and place them on the platter.</li><li>Arrange the grilled vegetables, olives, crumbled feta cheese or dairy-free alternatives, and any optional additions around the bowls.</li><li>Place whole grain crackers or pita bread alongside the other ingredients for dipping and scooping.</li></ul>
3	<ul><li>Garnish the mezze platter with fresh herbs or a drizzle of olive oil for added flavor and presentation.</li><li>Serve the mezze platter immediately as a colorful and flavorful appetizer or light meal.</li></ul>
4	<ul><li>Invite guests to gather around the mezze platter and enjoy the variety of flavors and textures.</li><li>Encourage them to mix and match different components to create their own flavor combinations.</li></ul>

Chapter 6: Dinner Recipes

Venison Stir-Fry with Broccoli and Bell Peppers

Preparation Time:	30 minutes

Ingredients

- 1 lb venison steak, thinly sliced
- 2 tablespoons soy sauce
- 1 tablespoon rice vinegar
- 1 tablespoon honey or maple syrup
- 2 cloves garlic, minced
- 1 teaspoon grated ginger
- 1 tablespoon vegetable oil
- 2 cups broccoli florets
- 1 bell pepper, sliced
- Cooked rice or noodles, for serving
- Optional garnish: sliced green onions, sesame seeds

Instructions

1. In a bowl, whisk together soy sauce, rice vinegar, honey or maple syrup, minced garlic, and grated

ginger. Add the thinly sliced venison steak to the marinade and let it marinate for at least 15 minutes.

2. Heat vegetable oil in a large skillet or wok over medium-high heat. Add the marinated venison steak and stir-fry for 2-3 minutes until browned.

3. Add the broccoli florets and sliced bell pepper to the skillet and continue stir-frying for another 3-4 minutes, or until the vegetables are tender-crisp and the venison is cooked to your desired doneness.

4. Serve the venison stir-fry hot over cooked rice or noodles, garnished with sliced green onions and sesame seeds if desired.

Seared Shrimp with Whole Grain Pilaf

Preparation Time:	20 minutes

Ingredients

- 1 lb wild-caught shrimp, peeled and deveined
- 2 tablespoons olive oil
- 2 cloves garlic, minced
- 1 teaspoon smoked paprika
- Salt and pepper to taste
- 2 cups cooked whole grain pilaf (such as quinoa, brown rice, or farro)

- Optional garnish: chopped fresh cilantro, lime wedges

Instructions

1	Heat olive oil in a large skillet over medium heat. Add minced garlic and cook until fragrant, about 1 minute.
2	Add the peeled and deveined shrimp to the skillet. Season with smoked paprika, salt, and pepper. Cook for 2-3 minutes per side, or until the shrimp are pink and opaque.
3	Serve the seared shrimp hot over cooked whole grain pilaf.
4	Garnish with chopped fresh cilantro and lime wedges before serving.

Chickpea and Tofu Curry over Brown Rice

| Preparation Time: | 45 minutes |

Ingredients

- 1 can (15 oz) chickpeas, drained and rinsed
- 1 block of tofu, cubed
- 2 tablespoons olive oil
- 1 onion, diced

- 2 cloves garlic, minced

- 1 tablespoon curry powder

- 1 teaspoon ground turmeric

- 1 can (14 oz) coconut milk

- Assorted vegetables (such as spinach, bell peppers, and cauliflower), chopped

- Cooked brown rice, for serving

- Optional garnish: chopped fresh cilantro, lime wedges

Instructions

1 Heat olive oil in a large skillet or saucepan over medium heat. Add diced onion and minced garlic, and sauté until softened, about 5 minutes.

2 Add chickpeas and cubed tofu to the skillet, along with curry powder and ground turmeric. Cook for 2-3 minutes, stirring occasionally.

3 Pour in the coconut milk and stir to combine. Bring the mixture to a simmer and cook for 10-15 minutes, or until the sauce has thickened slightly.

4 Add assorted chopped vegetables to the skillet and cook for an additional 5-7 minutes, or until the vegetables are tender.

5 Serve the chickpea and tofu curry hot over cooked brown rice.

| 6 | Garnish with chopped fresh cilantro and lime wedges, if desired. |

Chicken and Vegetable Stir-Fry

| Preparation Time: | 20 minutes |

Ingredients

- 1 lb boneless, skinless chicken breasts, thinly sliced
- 2 tablespoons soy sauce or tamari
- 1 tablespoon sesame oil
- 1 tablespoon vegetable oil
- 2 cloves garlic, minced
- 1 teaspoon grated ginger
- Assorted vegetables (such as bell peppers, broccoli, carrots, and snap peas), sliced
- Cooked rice or noodles, for serving
- Optional garnish: chopped green onions, sesame seeds

Instructions

| 1 | In a bowl, marinate the thinly sliced chicken breasts in soy sauce or tamari and sesame oil for 10-15 minutes. |

2	Heat vegetable oil in a large skillet or wok over medium-high heat. Add minced garlic and grated ginger, and sauté until fragrant, about 1 minute.
3	Add the marinated chicken slices to the skillet and stir-fry until cooked through, about 5-7 minutes.
4	Add assorted sliced vegetables to the skillet and stir-fry for an additional 3-5 minutes, or until they are tender-crisp.
5	Serve the chicken and vegetable stir-fry hot over cooked rice or noodles.
6	Garnish with chopped green onions and sesame seeds, if desired.

Sheet Pan Chicken Thighs with Potatoes and Seasonal Vegetables

Preparation Time:	40 minutes

Ingredients

- 4 bone-in, skin-on chicken thighs
- 4 medium potatoes, diced
- Assorted seasonal vegetables (such as carrots, bell peppers, zucchini, and cherry tomatoes), chopped

- 2 tablespoons olive oil

- 2 cloves garlic, minced

- 1 teaspoon dried thyme

- 1 teaspoon dried rosemary

- Salt and pepper to taste

- Optional garnish: chopped fresh parsley

Instructions

1	Preheat the oven to 425°F (220°C). Line a large sheet pan with parchment paper or aluminum foil for easy cleanup.
2	In a small bowl, combine olive oil, minced garlic, dried thyme, dried rosemary, salt, and pepper.
3	Place the diced potatoes and assorted seasonal vegetables on the prepared sheet pan. Drizzle with half of the olive oil mixture and toss to coat evenly.
4	Arrange the chicken thighs on the sheet pan, skin side up. Brush the remaining olive oil mixture over the chicken thighs.
5	Roast in the preheated oven for 25-30 minutes, or until the chicken is golden brown and cooked through, and the vegetables are tender.
6	Remove from the oven and let rest for a few minutes before serving.

| 7 | Serve the sheet pan chicken thighs with potatoes and seasonal vegetables hot, garnished with chopped fresh parsley if desired. |

Chicken and Quinoa Pilaf

| Preparation Time: | 30 minutes |

Ingredients

- 1 lb boneless, skinless chicken breasts, cubed
- 1 cup quinoa, rinsed
- 1 onion, diced
- 2 cloves garlic, minced
- 2 cups chicken broth
- 1 teaspoon dried thyme
- Salt and pepper to taste
- Optional garnish: chopped fresh parsley

Instructions

1	Set the Instant Pot to "Sauté" mode and heat olive oil. Add diced onion and minced garlic, and sauté until softened, about 5 minutes.
2	Add cubed chicken breasts and cook until browned, about 5 minutes.
3	Stir in rinsed quinoa, chicken broth, dried thyme, salt, and pepper.

4	Close the Instant Pot lid and set to "Manual" mode for 8 minutes.
5	Once the cooking time is complete, allow for a natural pressure release for 10 minutes, then carefully quick-release any remaining pressure.
6	Open the lid and fluff the quinoa pilaf with a fork. If desired, garnish with chopped fresh parsley before serving.

Mediterranean Turkey Skillet

Preparation Time:	25 minutes

Ingredients

- 1 lb ground turkey
- 1 onion, diced
- 2 cloves garlic, minced
- 1 bell pepper, diced
- 1 can (14 oz) diced tomatoes
- 1/2 cup sliced black olives
- 1 teaspoon dried oregano
- 1 teaspoon dried basil
- Salt and pepper to taste
- Optional garnish: crumbled feta cheese, chopped fresh parsley

Instructions

1. In a large skillet, cook ground turkey over medium heat until browned, breaking it apart with a spoon as it cooks.

2. Add diced onion, minced garlic, and diced bell pepper to the skillet, and cook until softened, about 5 minutes.

3. Stir in diced tomatoes (with juices), sliced black olives, dried oregano, dried basil, salt, and pepper. Cook for another 5-7 minutes, until heated through.

4. Serve the Mediterranean turkey skillet hot, garnished with crumbled feta cheese and chopped fresh parsley if desired.

Savory Seaweed Snack

Preparation Time:	20 minutes

Ingredients

- Ingredients:
- Nori sheets
- Sesame oil
- Soy sauce or tamari
- Chili flakes (optional)
- Salt (optional)

Instructions

1	Lay out the nori sheets on a flat surface.
2	<ul><li>Brush each nori sheet lightly with sesame oil to coat evenly.</li><li>Drizzle soy sauce or tamari over the nori sheets, spreading it evenly with a brush or the back of a spoon.</li><li>Sprinkle chili flakes over the seasoned nori sheets for a spicy kick, if desired.</li><li>Optionally, sprinkle a pinch of salt over the nori sheets for added flavor.</li></ul>

3	<ul><li>Preheat the oven to 250°F (120°C) or set a toaster oven to the lowest setting.</li><li>Place the seasoned nori sheets on a baking sheet lined with parchment paper or directly on the toaster oven rack.</li><li>Bake or toast the nori sheets for about 10-15 minutes until they become crispy and slightly curled up at the edges.</li></ul>
4	<ul><li>Allow the savory seaweed snacks to cool for a few minutes before serving.</li><li>Once cooled, break the nori sheets into smaller pieces or cut them into bite-sized squares using kitchen scissors.</li><li>Serve the savory seaweed snacks as a crunchy and satisfying snack option for any time of the day.</li></ul>

Protein-Packed Energy Bites

Preparation Time:	15 minutes

Ingredients

- 1 cup rolled oats
- 1/2 cup almond butter (or any nut butter of choice)
- 1/4 cup honey or maple syrup
- 2 tablespoons chia seeds
- 1/4 cup dark chocolate chips
- 1 teaspoon vanilla extract (optional)
- Pinch of salt (optional)
- Additional add-ins such as chopped nuts, dried fruit, or coconut flakes (optional)

Instructions

1.
   - In a large mixing bowl, combine rolled oats, almond butter, honey or maple syrup, chia seeds, dark chocolate chips, vanilla extract, and a pinch of salt (if using).
   - Stir until all ingredients are well combined and the mixture starts to come together. If the mixture seems too dry, add a bit more almond butter or honey/maple syrup.

2	<ul><li>Once the mixture is well combined, use a tablespoon to scoop out portions of the mixture.</li><li>Roll each portion between your palms to form into bite-sized balls.</li><li>If desired, roll the energy bites in additional add-ins such as chopped nuts, dried fruit, or coconut flakes for extra flavor and texture.</li></ul>
3	<ul><li>Place the energy bites on a baking sheet lined with parchment paper or a plate.</li><li>Chill the energy bites in the refrigerator for at least 30 minutes to firm up and hold their shape.</li></ul>
4	<ul><li>Once chilled, the protein-packed energy bites are ready to enjoy!</li><li>Store any leftover energy bites in an airtight container in the refrigerator for up to one week, or freeze for longer storage.</li></ul>

Homemade Veggie Chips

Preparation Time:	30 minutes

Ingredients

- 2 medium sweet potatoes
- 2 medium beets
- 1 bunch kale
- 2 tablespoons olive oil
- 1 teaspoon garlic powder
- 1 teaspoon paprika
- 1/2 teaspoon sea salt
- Optional: additional herbs and spices such as rosemary, thyme, or chili powder

Instructions

1	Preheat the oven to 325°F (160°C) and line two baking sheets with parchment paper.
2	• Wash and peel the sweet potatoes and beets. Using a mandoline slicer or a sharp knife, slice the sweet potatoes and beets into thin, uniform slices. • Wash the kale leaves and remove the stems. Tear the kale leaves into bite-sized pieces, discarding any tough stems.

3	<ul><li>In a large bowl, toss the sweet potato slices, beet slices, and kale pieces with olive oil until evenly coated.</li><li>Sprinkle the garlic powder, paprika, sea salt, and any additional herbs and spices over the vegetables. Toss again to coat evenly.</li></ul>
4	Arrange the seasoned veggie slices in a single layer on the prepared baking sheets, making sure they are not overlapping.
5	Bake the veggie chips in the preheated oven for 15-20 minutes, or until the edges are crispy and slightly golden brown. Keep an eye on them to prevent burning.
6	<ul><li>Remove the baking sheets from the oven and let the veggie chips cool for a few minutes before serving.</li><li>Once cooled, transfer the veggie chips to a serving bowl or store them in an airtight container for later enjoyment.</li></ul>

Frozen Yogurt Parfait Pops

Preparation Time:	10 minutes (plus freezing time)

Ingredients

- Greek yogurt (blood type O-friendly)
- Fresh fruit (such as berries, sliced bananas, or diced mango)
- Granola
- Honey or maple syrup (optional)
- Popsicle molds
- Popsicle sticks

Instructions

1
- Begin by spooning a layer of Greek yogurt into the bottom of each popsicle mold, filling them about one-third full.
- Add a layer of fresh fruit on top of the yogurt. You can use a single type of fruit or mix and match for variety.
- Sprinkle a layer of granola over the fruit. This adds crunch and texture to the popsicles.
- Repeat the layers until the popsicle molds are filled, alternating between yogurt, fruit, and granola. Leave a small space at the top of each mold for expansion during freezing.

2	Once the molds are filled, insert a popsicle stick into the center of each mold, making sure it stands upright.
3	Place the filled popsicle molds in the freezer and allow them to freeze until solid, usually for at least 4-6 hours or overnight.
4	Once the Frozen Yogurt Parfait Pops are frozen solid, remove them from the molds by running warm water over the outside of the molds for a few seconds to loosen the popsicles. Gently pull on the popsicle sticks to release the popsicles from the molds. Serve the Frozen Yogurt Parfait Pops immediately and enjoy this refreshing and protein-rich snack on hot summer days.

Dark Chocolate Truffles

Preparation Time:	20 minutes

Ingredients

- 1 cup pitted dates
- 1 cup almonds
- 3 tablespoons cocoa powder
- Shredded coconut or crushed nuts for rolling (optional)

Instructions

1	• If the dates are not already pitted, remove the pits and chop them into smaller pieces. • In a food processor, pulse the almonds until finely ground. Set aside.
2	• Add the chopped dates to the food processor and pulse until they form a sticky paste. • Add the ground almonds and cocoa powder to the date paste in the food processor. • Process the mixture until well combined and a thick, dough-like consistency forms.
3	• Scoop out small portions of the truffle mixture using a tablespoon or small cookie scoop. • Roll each portion between your palms to form a smooth ball. • If desired, roll the truffles in shredded coconut or crushed nuts for an extra layer of flavor and texture.
4	• Place the rolled truffles on a baking sheet lined with parchment paper. • Chill the truffles in the refrigerator for at least 30 minutes to firm up.

Avocado Chocolate Mousse Cups

Preparation Time:	15 minutes

Ingredients

- 2 ripe avocados, peeled and pitted
- 1/4 cup cocoa powder
- 1/4 cup honey or maple syrup
- 1 teaspoon vanilla extract
- Pinch of salt
- Optional toppings: whipped cream, berries, shaved chocolate

Instructions

1
- In a food processor or blender, combine the ripe avocados, cocoa powder, honey or maple syrup, vanilla extract, and a pinch of salt.
- Blend the ingredients until smooth and creamy, scraping down the sides of the blender as needed to ensure thorough mixing.

2
- Transfer the avocado chocolate mousse to a bowl or individual serving cups.
- Cover the mousse with plastic wrap, ensuring the plastic wrap touches the surface of the mousse to prevent any air from getting in.

	• Refrigerate the mousse for at least 1 hour to chill and allow the flavors to meld together.
3	• Once chilled, remove the avocado chocolate mousse from the refrigerator.
	• Serve the mousse in individual cups or bowls, garnished with optional toppings such as whipped cream, fresh berries, or shaved chocolate.
	• Enjoy this guilt-free dessert option with friends and family, savoring every creamy and decadent spoonful!
4	

Crispy Kale Popcorn

Preparation Time:	15 minutes (+ baking time)

Ingredients

- 1 bunch kale, washed and thoroughly dried
- 1 tablespoon olive oil
- 2 tablespoons nutritional yeast
- 1 teaspoon garlic powder
- 1/2 teaspoon paprika
- Salt and pepper to taste

Instructions

1	Preheat your oven to 300°F (150°C). Line a baking sheet with parchment paper or a silicone baking mat.
2	<ul><li>Remove the tough stems from the kale leaves and tear the leaves into bite-sized pieces.</li><li>Ensure the kale leaves are thoroughly dried using a salad spinner or paper towels. Moisture will prevent them from getting crispy.</li></ul>
3	<ul><li>Place the kale pieces in a large mixing bowl. Drizzle with olive oil and use your hands to massage the oil evenly into the kale leaves.</li><li>In a small bowl, mix together the nutritional yeast, garlic powder, paprika, salt, and pepper. Sprinkle the seasoning mixture over the kale and toss until the leaves are coated evenly.</li></ul>
4	Arrange the seasoned kale leaves in a single layer on the prepared baking sheet, ensuring they are not overlapping.
5	<ul><li>Place the baking sheet in the preheated oven and bake the kale for 10-15 minutes, or until the edges are crispy and lightly browned.</li><li>Keep an eye on the kale towards the end of the baking time to prevent burning.</li></ul>

<table>
<tr><td>6</td><td>

- Once crispy, remove the kale popcorn from the oven and let them cool on the baking sheet for a few minutes.
- Transfer the crispy kale popcorn to a serving bowl and enjoy immediately as a savory and nutritious snack!

</td></tr>
</table>

Nutty Banana Bread Bites

Preparation Time:	15 minutes (+ baking time)

Ingredients

- 2 ripe bananas, mashed
- 1 cup almond flour
- 1/4 cup chopped nuts (such as walnuts or pecans)
- 2 tablespoons honey or maple syrup
- 1 teaspoon vanilla extract
- 1/2 teaspoon cinnamon
- 1/4 teaspoon baking soda
- Pinch of salt

Instructions

1 Preheat your oven to 350°F (175°C). Grease a mini muffin tin or line it with paper liners.

2 In a mixing bowl, combine the mashed bananas, almond flour, chopped nuts, honey or maple syrup,

vanilla extract, cinnamon, baking soda, and a pinch of salt. Stir until well combined.

3 Spoon the batter evenly into the prepared mini muffin tin, filling each cup nearly to the top.

4 Place the muffin tin in the preheated oven and bake the banana bread bites for 12-15 minutes, or until golden brown and a toothpick inserted into the center comes out clean.

5
- Once baked, remove the muffin tin from the oven and let the banana bread bites cool in the tin for a few minutes.
- Transfer the bites to a wire rack to cool completely before serving.

6
- Enjoy the nutty banana bread bites as a delicious and nutritious snack any time of day.
- Store any leftovers in an airtight container at room temperature for up to 3 days, or freeze for longer storage.

Chapter 8: Integrating Exercise and Lifestyle Practices

Exercise Recommendations for Blood Type O Individuals

Blood type O individuals are often described as the "hunter-gatherers" of human evolution, with ancestors who thrived on high-protein diets and regular physical activity. As a result, blood type O individuals tend to have robust metabolisms and a natural inclination towards physical exertion.

Blood type O individuals typically excel in activities that require strength, endurance, and agility. They may have a higher proportion of fast-twitch muscle fibers, making them well-suited for activities like sprinting, weightlifting, and martial arts. Additionally, blood type O individuals may benefit from exercise that stimulates the production of dopamine and endorphins, such as high-intensity interval training (HIIT) and outdoor activities.

Recommended Exercise Modalities:

1. Strength Training: Incorporate regular strength training sessions into your exercise routine to build and maintain lean muscle mass. Focus on compound exercises like squats, deadlifts, bench presses, and pull-ups, which engage multiple muscle groups simultaneously. Aim for moderate to heavy resistance and perform 2-3 sets of 8-12 repetitions per exercise.

2. High-Intensity Interval Training (HIIT): HIIT workouts are highly effective for blood type O individuals, as they can boost metabolism, improve cardiovascular health, and increase fat burning in a short amount of time. Alternate between periods of high-intensity exercise (e.g., sprinting, jumping jacks, burpees) and active recovery (e.g., walking, jogging) for a total of 20-30 minutes.

3. Cardiovascular Exercise: Incorporate cardiovascular exercise into your routine to improve heart health and endurance. Opt for activities that you enjoy and that align with your preferences and lifestyle, such as running, cycling, swimming, or hiking. Aim for at least 150 minutes of moderate-intensity cardio or 75 minutes of vigorous-intensity cardio per week.

4. Flexibility and Mobility Training: Don't overlook the importance of flexibility and mobility training for blood type O individuals. Incorporate stretching exercises, yoga, or Pilates into your routine to improve joint mobility, prevent injury, and promote relaxation and stress relief. Focus on dynamic stretches that engage multiple muscle groups and movements.

5. Outdoor Activities: Take advantage of outdoor activities that align with your natural inclination towards physical exertion. Activities like hiking, trail running, rock climbing, and obstacle courses can provide a challenging workout while connecting you with nature and reducing stress levels.

Tailoring Your Exercise Routine:

As with any exercise program, it's essential to tailor your routine to your individual preferences, abilities, and goals. Listen to your body and adjust your workouts accordingly, taking into account factors like recovery time, sleep quality, and overall stress levels. Consult with a fitness professional or healthcare provider if you have any underlying health conditions or concerns.

21-day Week Exercise Routine

Week 1: Establishing the Foundation

Day 1	20 minutes of brisk walking or jogging
	10 minutes of bodyweight exercises (squats, lunges, push-ups)
	5 minutes of stretching and cooldown
Day 2	30 minutes of low-impact cardio (cycling, swimming, elliptical)
	10 minutes of core exercises (planks, Russian twists, bicycle crunches)
	5 minutes of stretching and cooldown
Day 3	Rest day or gentle yoga/stretching session for recovery
Day 4	20 minutes of interval training (alternating between bursts of high-intensity exercise and periods of rest)
	10 minutes of resistance training (dumbbell squats, bicep curls, tricep dips)
	5 minutes of stretching and cooldown
Day 5	30 minutes of moderate-intensity cardio (brisk walking, jogging)
	10 minutes of bodyweight exercises focusing on lower body (lunges, squats, calf raises)

	5 minutes of stretching and cooldown
Day 6	Rest day or active recovery such as hiking or gentle swimming
Day 7	40 minutes of low-impact cardio (cycling, swimming)
	15 minutes of full-body strength training using resistance bands or bodyweight exercises
	10 minutes of stretching and cooldown
Week 2: Increasing Intensity	
Day 1	20 minutes of interval training (sprinting, jumping jacks, burpees)
	15 minutes of core exercises (planks, mountain climbers, leg raises)
	5 minutes of stretching and cooldown
Day 2	30 minutes of cardio (running, cycling, rowing)
	15 minutes of upper body strength training (push-ups, shoulder presses, rows)
	5 minutes of stretching and cooldown
Day 3	Rest day or gentle yoga/stretching session for recovery
Day 4	25 minutes of circuit training (alternating between cardio and strength exercises)
	15 minutes of lower body strength training (squats, deadlifts, lunges)

	5 minutes of stretching and cooldown
Day 5	30 minutes of high-intensity interval training (HIIT) incorporating bodyweight exercises and plyometrics
	10 minutes of core exercises (crunches, Russian twists, plank variations)
	5 minutes of stretching and cooldown
Day 6	Rest day or active recovery such as swimming or cycling at a leisurely pace
Day 7	45 minutes of steady-state cardio (brisk walking, jogging, cycling)
	20 minutes of full-body strength training using weights or resistance bands
	10 minutes of stretching and cooldown
Week 3: Consolidating Gains	
Day 1	30 minutes of interval training (sprinting, jumping jacks, mountain climbers)
	15 minutes of core exercises (planks, bicycle crunches, leg raises)
	5 minutes of stretching and cooldown
Day 2	40 minutes of moderate-intensity cardio (running, cycling)
	20 minutes of upper body strength training (push-ups, dumbbell rows, shoulder presses)

	5 minutes of stretching and cooldown
Day 3	Rest day or gentle yoga/stretching session for recovery
Day 4	30 minutes of circuit training (incorporating a mix of cardio and strength exercises)
	20 minutes of lower body strength training (squats, lunges, deadlifts)
	5 minutes of stretching and cooldown
Day 5	35 minutes of high-intensity interval training (HIIT) with emphasis on explosive movements and plyometrics
	15 minutes of core exercises (planks, Russian twists, leg raises)
	5 minutes of stretching and cooldown
Day 6	Rest day or active recovery such as hiking or swimming
Day 7	50 minutes of steady-state cardio (brisk walking, jogging, cycling)
	25 minutes of full-body strength training using weights or resistance bands
	10 minutes of stretching and cooldown

Conclusion

In conclusion, the journey towards embracing the Blood Type O diet and meal plan is a deeply personal and transformative experience. Throughout this book, we've delved into the intricacies of understanding blood type O, exploring its genetic implications, and uncovering the unique characteristics and health implications associated with it.

We've outlined the principles of the Blood Type O diet, emphasizing the importance of embracing certain foods while avoiding others to optimize health and well-being. From meal planning basics to sample meal plans tailored to various lifestyles, we've provided practical guidance for incorporating these principles into everyday life.

Moreover, we've gone beyond static meal plans, advocating for a seasonal rotation approach and strategic meal pairing to enhance nutrient absorption and energy levels. By encouraging creativity and flexibility in meal preparation, we empower readers to cultivate a deeper connection with their food and nourish their bodies in alignment with their blood type.

In addition to meal planning, we've explored the importance of regular exercise, stress management techniques, and strategies for navigating social events and dining out successfully. By addressing these holistic aspects of health, we support readers in achieving balance and vitality in all areas of their lives.

Throughout the journey, it's crucial to celebrate successes and milestones, no matter how small, and to approach setbacks with resilience and determination. By maintaining consistency, cultivating self-awareness, and fostering a positive mindset, individuals can empower themselves to thrive on their health journey.

As we conclude this book, let us remember that embracing the Blood Type O diet is not just about following a set of rules but about embracing a lifestyle rooted in self-care, nourishment, and vitality. May this knowledge serve as a guide and inspiration as you embark on your own journey towards optimal health and well-being.

www.ingramcontent.com/pod-product-compliance
Lightning Source LLC
Chambersburg PA
CBHW050823250726
48653CB00006B/2390